TRANSLATIONAL MEDICINE,
DIABETES AND METABOLIC SYNDROME X:
The story of how dolphins defeat diabetes and more......

Stephen Holt, MD
www.stephenholtmd.com

BOOK DATA

Holt Institute of Medicine, 2016

25 Amity Street, Little Falls, New Jersey 07424

Tel.: 973-256-4660

Email: drholt@hiom.org

ISBN: 978-0-9972643-0-2

Printed in the United States of America

Published by the Holt Institute of Medicine and Create Space Publishing Platform, 2016

Cover image by Mark Interrante.

KEY WORDS: 1. Diabetes Mellitus 2. Metabolic Syndrome 3. Syndrome X 4. Dolphin research 5. Heptadecanoic acid 6. Saturated fat 7. Trans-fats 8. Dietary Supplementation 9. Translational research.

CONTENTS

PREFACE

STEPHEN HOLT MD

Diabetes affects more than 26 million Americans, but a pre-diabetic state occurs in about 83 million adult Americans in the form of Metabolic Syndrome X, or what has been called pre-diabetes. This diabetic and pre-diabetic epidemic accounts for the expenditure of many billions of dollars of medical interventions per annum, but no cure exists. The absence of a cure for diabetes is related to the fact that the root cause of this modern medical epidemic remains unknown. This book speculates that findings in marine mammals on a switch away from diabetic-like states may be relevant to the cause of diabetes and Metabolic Syndrome X in humans

The scientific observation that dolphins can defeat diabetes has been linked to their diet that may include a special type of saturated dietary fat. This fat is called (heptadecanoic acid, (C-17). These findings that implicate heptadecanoic acid in the prevention of diabetes-like states are the result of ground-breaking research that was performed at the National Marine Mammal Foundation (NMMF). This booklet recounts these recent observations and it is written in a format to be easily understood by the lay person. In addition, these findings shed preliminary light for healthcare professionals on what may be one of the most important modern discoveries of the potential cause of diabetes mellitus and Metabolic Syndrome X.

This short book describes intriguing research on dolphins who are known to develop the important forerunner to diabetes known as Metabolic Syndrome X and "diabetes-like states" (pre-diabetes). The proposals are simple and focus on the fact that a saturated fat called heptadecanoic acid (C-17:0 or margaric acid) may be deficient in the diet of certain dolphins. This deficiency is believed to lead to the development of Metabolic Syndrome X or prediabetes or diabetes-like states. This book presents evidence that justifies the extrapolation to humans of a deficiency of heptadecanoic acid (C-17). This saturated fatty acid deficiency may be a cause of diabetes, Metabolic Syndrome X and some of their sequelae in humans. Supplementation of this saturated fatty acid (C-17, heptadecanoic acid) in dolphins reverses the diabetes-like status of dolphins and ameliorates the associated laboratory indicators of the occurrence of Metabolic Syndrome X in these mammals. Whether or not the same situation exists in humans requires verification in future research.

By inference and with promising supportive evidence, heptadecanoic acid (C-17, margaric acid) may be a root cause of diabetes in humans, where it is known that the presence of this saturated fat is correlated (associated) with reductions in coronary heart disease (CHD). In turn, it is known that coronary heart disease is associated with Metabolic Syndrome X and diabetes mellitus.

For about forty years there has been a focus on low fat diets for health, with a number of positive claims for cardiovascular health and diabetes prevention. That said, the scientific foundations to promote the widespread adoption of low fat diets has been questioned repeatedly, especially in recent times. Contemporary studies start to question the lack of prudence of low fat diets to promote general health. While recommendations for a low saturated fat diet persist in official American Dietary Guidelines (2016), no limits have been placed on dietary cholesterol intake in otherwise healthy people.

Findings in both dolphin and human research have kindled a modern revolution in thought about the wisdom (or lack thereof) of the low fat diet. These findings have been projected to humans with the idea that there may be a benefit from the dietary inclusion of certain saturated fats, notably heptadecanoic acid. Heptadecanoic acid is present in whole fat dairy foods (butter and whole fat yogurt), rye, animal fat and shark liver oil. Switching diets toward inclusion of extra saturated fat may not be an attractive option for some people and not all saturated fats in the diet have been considered to be desirable for health. However, hexadecanoic acid can be administered by a change of diet or with greater ease in a simple dietary supplement format. By inference, this fatty acid can be combined with other nutrients to provide support for prediabetic management (Metabolic Syndrome X) or for their potential benefit in the management of diabetes mellitus, e.g. alpha lipoic acid.

The notion that "Dolphins Defeat Diabetes" seems to be a long way from diabetes prevention in humans, but the translational medical science linking these circumstances to humans appears quite strong. The correction of any deficiencies of heptadecanoic acid (C-17:0, margaric acid) in the diet may have emerged with many putative health advantages and it is consistent with the idea that certain fatty acids play unique and specific metabolic roles. Many fatty acids are essential and they cannot be synthesized by the human body. In this context, taking heptadecanoic acid appears to be akin to using a necessary "vitamin supplement" and it has promise as a safe way of potentially providing insurance against Metabolic Syndrome X, prediabetes and perhaps type 11diabetes mellitus.

The circumstances have been summarized in an eloquent manner by one of the lead researchers in the field, Dr. Stephanie Venn-Watson (of the NMMF) who has associated the findings in Dolphin research with human circumstances and stated the following. *"We hypothesize that widespread movement away from whole fat dairy products in humans may have created unanticipated heptadecanoic acid (C-17) deficiencies and in turn, this dietary deficiency may be playing a role in the global diabetes pandemic". Many individuals are* anxiously awaiting a filling-in of the gaps of reasoning on translational research from dolphins to humans.

Stephen Holt, MD
Little Falls, New Jersey, 2016
www.stephenholtmd.com

FOREWORD

JOHN SALERNO D.O.

This book tells a powerful scientific story about how saturated fat (dairy) with its content of heptadecanoic acid (C-17.0, margaric acid) may assist in the prevention and even the treatment of Metabolic Syndrome X and diabetes mellitus. In my work with the late Dr. Robert Atkins there were constant questions and doubts about the espoused benefits of the low fat diet. Proponents of the low fat diet have claimed that the low carb, high fat dietary approach is unhealthy or even dangerous. The tide now appears to be starting to turn!

In these writings, Dr. Holt focuses on the interesting observations of the National Marine Mammal Foundation (NMMF) where dolphins may develop diabetes mellitus, Metabolic Syndrome X or a diabetes-like state. This status in dolphins can be reversed by the application of dietary supplementation with the saturated fat heptadecanoic acid (C-17, margaric acid). Dr. Holt proposes that the benefits of heptadecanoic acid supplementation can be beneficial in humans with Metabolic Syndrome X or diabetes and these desirable effects may be amplified by the co-administration of alpha-lipoic acid (a powerful antioxidant compound) or other anti-diabetic nutraceuticals. There has been much learned from the study of marine life and its potential impact in humans. Maybe the notion that "Dolphins Defeat Diabetes" will provide a pivotal basis to prevent diabetes?

This book is novel, short and to the point. The recent rethinking of the shallow benefits, if any, of a low fat diet are highlighted in a thoughtful manner by Dr. Holt. A simple issue of major importance is raised in this book. If fat is reduced in the diet, calories are sourced often from increasing carbohydrate intake. In fact, much of the increasing weight gain of the nation in recent years has occurred as a consequence of increase carbohydrate intake, not as a result of fat intake.

The vilification of saturated fat in the diet has been argued for years. It is gratifying to see that there has been a change in American Dietary Guidelines

(2016) to move away from some unsubstantiated facts that a low fat/low cholesterol diet is necessarily a generic promoter of general health.

This book is a must read and it presents new, novel and exciting findings on potential nutritional solutions to Metabolic Syndrome X and diabetes mellitus.

John Salerno, DO
www.salernocenter.com
New York, New York, 2016

INTRODUCTION

Diabetes mellitus is the focus of a widespread epidemic on a global basis. It is a major public health problem with a 41 percent increase in its occurrence since 2007 (according to the American Diabetes Association). Scientific experts refer to diabetes as a pandemic (severe epidemic) in the U.S.A. and it affects more than 26 million Americans. Future projections of the occurrence of diabetes mellitus are staggering. There are estimates, based on current trends, that diabetes mellitus may affect one in three adults by the year 2050.

Diabetes mellitus is classified in simple terms as Type 1 diabetes, previously referred to as juvenile diabetes, and the more common Type 11 diabetes, often called maturity onset diabetes. Type 11 diabetes accounts for approximately 90 percent of all cases of diabetes and it is often preceded by a condition called Metabolic Syndrome X or prediabetes. In Metabolic Syndrome the variable occurrence of high blood sugar, blood cholesterol and blood pressure are linked by the presence of resistance to the actions of the hormone insulin. Insulin is the principal hormone that controls blood sugar. In brief, the simple definition of Metabolic Syndrome X includes a high blood sugar (with or without high blood cholesterol and or high blood pressure) and 40 inch plus waist size in men or 35 inches in women (obesity). While there have been many advances in the management of diabetes or Metabolic Syndrome X, the root causes of these disorders remain unknown and a cure does not exist for these conditions. It should be emphasized that discussions about diabetes prevention in this book are relevant to type 11 diabetes, not to type 1 diabetes.

This monograph describes a newly discovered finding by researchers at the National Marine Mammal Foundation NMMF) that dolphins (marine mammals) can control Metabolic Syndrome X (Syndrome X) as a consequence of increasing their dietary intake of a special type of saturated dietary fat called heptadecanoic (or C-17). Moreover, it has been demonstrated that a deficiency of this fat is associated with the development of a prediabetic or diabetic-like state in dolphins (*PLOS ONE, July 22, 2015. DOI 101371/journal pone 0132117 and www.medicalexpress.com/news/2015-07-dolphins-diabetes-humans.html*).

Much of the novel research described in this short book has been performed by the National Marine Mammal Foundation (NMMF), specifically Dr. Stephanie Venn-Watson (Director of NMMF's Translational Medicine Research Program) and her colleagues (*Venn-Watson S. K. et al Increased Dietary Intake of Saturated Fatty Acid Heptadecanoic (C-17:0) Associated with Decreasing Ferritin and Alleviated Metabolic Syndrome in Dolphins PLOS ONE, 2015; 10(7): e0132117 DOI; 10, 1371/journal pone 0132117*). These studies have been described as relevant to humans to provide a potential explanation that an increase in Type 11 diabetes and Metabolic Syndrome X may be due to a lack of specific saturated fats in the diet (notably C-17, heptadecanoic acid).

THE PRINCIPAL RESEARCH FINDINGS PRESENT A HYPOTHESIS

Both captive and wild dolphins can develop Metabolic Syndrome X (prediabetes) and they are able to switch in and out of a prediabetic or diabetic-like state. This intriguing phenomenon appears to be related to both fasting and the presence of certain dietary factors (notably the saturated fatty acid, C-17). The National Marine Foundation researchers examined the fatty acid levels in the blood of dolphins and, at the same time, looked at the fatty acid levels in their fish diet. The surprising finding in these studies of 55 different fatty acids was that the C-17 saturated fat, known as heptadecanoic acid, appeared to have the most beneficial effect on the dolphin's body biochemistry (metabolism). It was found that heptadecanoic acid appeared to reverse Metabolic Syndrome X and a diabetes-like state in dolphins .

In these studies (*Venn-Watson S K et ibid, 2015*), it appeared that the dolphins with the highest levels of heptadecanoic acid (C17) had lower markers of Metabolic Syndrome (Syndrome X) with notable reductions in blood triglyceride and insulin levels. In Metabolic Syndrome these markers are often high and are major hallmarks of the presence of this disorder of body metabolism. In addition, the studies of fatty acid content of the dietary fish of the dolphins showed variable amounts of heptadecanoic acid (C-17:0, margaric acid). In some cases there were negligible amounts of C-17 (heptadecanoic acid) in some dietary fish consumed by the dolphins, whereas certain dietary fish had very high levels of C-17, (notably mullet and mackerel fish).

To further examine this relationship between the presence of heptadecanoic acid and the amelioration of Metabolic Syndrome X, six dolphins were fed fish diets that were high in heptadecanoic acid (C-17). About six months following the institution of the high C-17 diet, favorable effects on markers of Metabolic Syndrome X were noted with a reduction of elevated insulin levels (overcoming of insulin resistance). Moreover, blood glucose triglyceride and serum ferritin levels returned towards normal. Serum ferritin is known to be a detectable change that is a forerunner to Metabolic Syndrome X and type 11 diabetes mellitus.

METABOLIC SYNDROME IN HUMANS

As mentioned earlier, Syndrome X affects about 83 million Americans without widespread recognition of its presence, among its victims or their doctors. The term Syndrome X is applied to the variable combination of obesity, high blood cholesterol, poor blood glucose balance (insulin resistance) and high blood pressure. In its classic form, Syndrome X is characterized by the pot-bellied, fifty year-old person who worries about his or her blood cholesterol, whilst they are unaware of glucose intolerance due to insulin resistance. However, Syndrome X comes in many guises that share a common underlying feature of resistance to the actions of the hormone insulin. The constellation of disorders within Syndrome X aggregate together to kill or cripple many people in an insidious manner by creating a widespread risk for cardiovascular and other diseases. There is a defined role of insulin resistance in the cause of several other disorders including: female infertility, inflammatory disorders, immune impairment Alzheimer's disease and perhaps cancer.

The cause and effect relationships among the four cardinal components of Metabolic Syndrome X have become increasingly clear to modern science, largely as a consequence of the work of the eminent Stanford University physician, Dr. G. Reaven MD. Dr. Reaven coined the terms "Syndrome X" in 1988 to describe the interrelationship of obesity, high blood pressure and raised blood sugar (insulin resistance) with elevated blood cholesterol and blood triglycerides. There is clear evidence to incriminate "central types" of obesity and perhaps changes of protein metabolism with high blood uric acid within the syndrome. I have extended the description of the components of Syndrome X to support the notion of what I have termed Syndrome X, Y and Z.... where disease risks beyond cardiovascular problems emerge with clarity. The disorders within Syndrome X are inextricably linked with adverse lifestyle in a "bouquet of barbed wire" that is both killing Western nations and robbing them of health (*Holt S, Combat Syndrome X, Y and Z.... Wellness Publishing, 2002*).

There are about 26 million Americans with diabetes mellitus. Data imply that many do not know that they have it and there are many who have a "pre-diabetic state". As long ago as August 2001, the U.S. Secretary of Human Health and Social Services joined researchers from Harvard University and the National Institutes of Health to call for a major public health initiative to educate the US population on the prevention of diabetes mellitus (and related disorders that form Metabolic Syndrome X). These national proclamations, more than a decade ago, warned of the shocking increase in diabetes and pre-diabetic disorders in all age groups and presented clear evidence that weight loss and exercise helps to prevent these diseases. It is clear that Metabolic Syndrome X and type 11 diabetes are of multifactorial etiology (many causes).

RESEARCH AT THE NATIONAL MARINE MAMMAL FOUNDATION

The dolphin is a marine mammal that shares similarity with humans, especially because of brain size. Humans, primates and dolphins have the largest brain size among mammals and this makes the availability of glucose particularly important for the support of vital brain function. Dolphins do not eat sugar. Their diet is mainly composed of fish.

Dolphins can rapidly transport sugar on the red blood cells, like humans and primates. In common with humans, dolphins have obligatory needs to keep brain functioning optimal and this situation provides supplementary evidence for the importance of efficient mechanisms of glucose regulation in humans and dolphins.

As mentioned earlier, the NMMF has examined in detail how humans and dolphins are alike in their body structures and functions. The brains of dolphins and humans are relatively large in proportion to body size and parts of a dolphin's brain has even more folds than humans, allowing neurological activity (brain functions). Moreover, red blood cells of dolphins and humans can carry glucose which is absolutely necessary for brain function. In addition, dolphins and humans have other health challenges in common. For example, they share a number of similar diseases e.g. viral infections and certain fungal infections.

Humans with diabetes or Metabolic Syndrome X and dolphins have a tendency to store too much iron and fat in their livers (fatty liver). Dolphins with iron overload in their liver may have a disease called hemochromatosis (iron overload) and if they are fed high protein or sugar diets they get high levels of blood sugar that last for a period of five to ten hours. Dolphins with this kind of iron overload tend to have raised blood insulin levels (hyperinsulinemia) which is found often in type 11 diabetes and in many cases of Metabolic Syndrome X.

According to the National Marine Mammal Foundation (NMMF), dolphins have a "switch" that can turn diabetes on and off. Research at the NMMF is focused on the genetic, environmental and dietary factors of this "switch" with collaboration with the Salk Institute for Biological Studies. The hope is that these research pathways will help understand the management of diabetes-like, body metabolism in dolphins and find an avenue to treat and cure diabetes in humans.

In advanced studies at the NMMF, more than one thousand blood tests from dolphins were examined. These studies permitted assessments of blood sugar and other markers after an overnight fast and after eating. These blood tests showed that dolphins had blood values that were diabetes-like in the morning but not in the afternoon. The NMMF believes that finding the understanding that the mechanisms of this diabetes "switch" in dolphins could lead to the identification of a cure for diabetes in humans.

Clearly, the more recent findings of the role of heptadecanoic acid (C-17:0) in this switch from diabetes-like to normal body status is a pivotal finding in the research performed by the NMMF. Further details of these findings are available at *www.nmmf.org/diabetes/metabolism/*.

A CLOSER LOOK AT C-17 (heptadecanoic acid)

Heptadecanoic acid is sometimes called margaric acid or C-17:0 and it is found in certain fish, rye, dairy fat, beef fat and shark liver oil. C-17 (heptadecanoic acid) is a saturated fat. While everyone has heard of the health benefits of <u>unsaturated</u> fatty acids, for example, omega 3 fatty acids from fish oil or omega 6 fatty acids from plants, the presence of saturated fat in the diet has tended to be associated with chronic disease. This circumstance has led to four decades of the popularity of low fat diets and the intake of non-fat dairy products which do not contain any C-17 (heptadecanoic acid). However, the proposed benefits of low fat diets have been questioned, especially in contemporary medical literature – vide infra.

Stephanie Venn-Watson and her colleagues (from NMMF) have presented a hypothesis that the low-fat diet popularization could have created C-17 (heptadecanoic acid) deficiencies in humans; and that this may be an important factor in the widespread prevalence (occurrence) of diabetes mellitus. Of course, some scientists have started to challenge the link of diabetes development and C-17 deficiency by pointing out differences in how fat is handled and stored by dolphins. For example, dolphins have a functional blubber layer beneath their skin. That said, the pathways of fatty acid handling among different mammals (including dolphins and humans) share similarities. The president of the NMMF, Dr. Samuel Ridgway, has remarked that the dolphin studies involving C-17 appear to be an example of how improving the health of dolphins may be a pathway to benefit human health. This circumstance is a prime example of translational medical research.

Heptadecanoic acid belongs to a family of saturated, odd numbered fatty acid chains including: pentadecanoic acid, nonadecanoic acid, heneicosanoic acid and tricosanoic acid. Fatty acids with odd numbered carbon chains are often produced from the three carbon compound proprionic acid. Vitamin B_{12} facilitates the conversion of proprionic acid into succinic acid which becomes oxidized subsequently in energy pathways. Lack of vitamin B_{12} can cause a build up of odd numbered chain fatty acids. Bacteria in the gut of ruminants, (for example, sheep and cows) may produce large amounts of proprionate (proprionic acid) and it is possible theoretically that the human gut could produce substantial amounts of proprionate leading to an elevation of odd chain fatty acids. However, this latter circumstance is unlikely in humans, except in the presence of gut dysbiosis (upset of the bacterial inhabitants of the bowel). To my knowledge, there have been no studies in dolphins concerning these matters, but as mentioned, odd numbered fatty acids are produced by ruminant animals, e.g. cows.

GENETICS

Comparisons of human and dolphin genes (genetic make-up) that can affect the "diabetes switch" are underway. Researchers at the Salk Institute have located a "fasting gene" that is expressed in people with diabetes mellitus. Further studies in dolphins that determine how a fasting gene is turned on and off in dolphins may result in applied technology in humans to genetically control the sugar-handling process (*www.calacademy.org/explore-science/dolphins-Feb. 19, 2010, Science News "Dolphins and Diabetes"*) and (*Chowdhury R. et al Association of Dietary, Circulating, and Supplement Fatty Acids with Coronary Risk: A systematic Review and Meta-analysis 18 March, 2014, Vol. 160. No.6: 398-406.doi:10.7326/M13-1788*). Moreover, there is current evidence that does not support some of the dietary guidelines to encourage higher intake of polyunsaturated fatty acids and a lower intake of total saturated fats for the prevention of a variety of chronic diseases.

FUTURE STUDIES

Clearly, there are many future studies to perform, such as how changes in dietary fish sources for dolphins may occur with climatic or other environmental changes and how this could affect body metabolism in dolphins. Moreover, further human studies are required to test the effects of C-17 (heptadecanoic acid) supplementation on individuals with metabolic Syndrome X and to test the occurrence of C-17 deficiencies in prediabetic individuals.

The NMMF has announced its collaboration with children's' hospitals to attempt to examine levels of C-17 in youngsters with diabetes mellitus or Metabolic Syndrome. A number of senior researchers remain quite optimistic that C-17 may help reverse pre-diabetes and benefit diabetes mellitus in humans.

THE HIGH FAT, HIGH CHOLESTEROL DIET

There is an accumulation of scientific evidence that dietary cholesterol and saturated fat intake are not as damaging to health to a degree that has been proposed previously, in a widespread popular manner. It has been finally recognized in the new American Dietary Guidelimes (Jan. 2016) that most cholesterol comes from within the body as a consequence of body metabolism (synthesis of cholesterol). Dietary cholesterol makes a smaller contribution to blood cholesterol levels than its manufacture within the body. Moreover, dietary guidelines for a low saturated fat diet have been questioned in recent medical publications in the United Kingdom (BMJ), where it has been concluded that the low far guidelines are not supported consistently by conclusive research. For many years there has been a minority group of physicians who have espoused the benefits of selected saturated fats in the diet and their points of view are attracting renaissance interest.

Dr. Venn-Watson reinforced her hypothesis on the potential role of C-17 in diabetes prevention by stating *"We hypothesize that widespread movement away from whole fat dairy products in humans may have created unanticipated heptadecanoic acid (C-17) deficiencies, and in turn, this dietary deficiency may be playing a role in the global diabetes pandemic"* (quoted by *Hal Conick www.dairyreporter.com/Markets/Lack-ofdairy-based-fat-in-human-diet-mayleadto..., accessed 7/28/15*). Dr. Venn-Watson has pointed out that there are a number of studies performed in Europe and Japan that have linked higher blood levels of heptadecanoic acid (C-17) to a lower risk of Metabolic Syndrome X and Type 11 diabetes.

THE LOW FAT "CRAZE" IN MODERN PERSPECTIVE

Recent findings have indicated that dietary recommendations, introduced for more than 220 million Americans and 56 million United Kingdom citizens by the year 1983, were made on "shaky ground". In fact, there was an absence of supporting evidence from scientific studies (randomized controlled trials) to support these previous dietary guidelines. In an excellent review of this subject, Kurt Wood examines this issue (*Every last shred of evidence": Why low-fat dietary guidelines should never have been introduced www.diabetes.co.uk/in-depth/every-last-shred-evidence-low-fat-dietary-guidelines-..., accessed 7/28/2015*).

A pivotal medical publication emerged in June, 2015 (*Harcombe Z et al, the BMJ Open Heart Journal "Evidence from randomized controlled trials did not support the introduction of dietary fat guidelines in 1977 and 1983, a systematic review and metanalysis"*). This June, 2015 study provides a detailed critical account of the evidence originally used to support the low fat guidelines for diet that have been debated for about 40 years. In brief, the analysis of the body of recently reviewed scientific evidence did not find any relationship between dietary fat intake and deaths from coronary heart disease (CHD) or all causes, regardless of reductions in blood cholesterol levels (*Harcombe Z, ibid, 2015*). These findings have been used to question the role of elevated serum cholesterol levels in the development of CHD. Moreover, it argues against the belief that reducing dietary fat (saturated fat) causes a definitive reduction in CHD. Hence, the "high cholesterol high saturated fat theories" have been questioned by this modern research!

To make the point, the common idea that lowering cholesterol intake by lowering saturated fat intake can result in lower rates of heart disease is clearly in doubt. Thus, the notion of lowering dietary fat (saturated fat) intake to reduce the occurrence of heart disease may be somewhat of a fallacy, except perhaps in individuals with high blood cholesterol (LDL). A major scientific challenge to the implied wisdom of the low fat approach for the prevention of cardiovascular disease has come from the Danish Scientist Dr. Uffe Ravnskov. This researcher has drawn attention to several flawed clinical trials and epidemiological (population) studies that have propagated the misleading notion that high fat intake is harmful to human health and that reductions of fat intake may be advantageous for health.

Perhaps the best known recent protagonist of fat inclusion in the diet was Robert Atkins, MD (deceased) with his proposals in his best selling book "The Diet Revolution" and other writings. These proposals have been reinforced by contemporary authors such as Dr. John Salerno in his new book titled "Fight Fat with Fat". Some recent observations have shown the benefit of low carbohydrate diets in enhancing weight loss and improving HbA1c levels (a measure of diabetic control) in individuals with type 11 diabetes. These findings challenge positions on diet compositions for diabetics that have been adopted by some agencies for diabetes in the U.S.A. and Europe.

HEPTADECANOIC ACID AND A LOW OCCURRENCE OF HEART DISEASE

A study based on information from 72 unique population studies (with over 600,000 participants from 18 nations) was reported by Dr. Rajiv Chowdhury and colleagues, coordinated through the University of Cambridge in the United Kingdom. Dr. Chowdhury and his colleagues reported in this study that the presence of fatty acids did not appear to be associated with coronary heart disease (CHD). In particular, there appeared to be no link between heart health and the presence of polyunsaturated fatty acids (omega 3 and 6 unsaturated fatty acids).

The data in these studies showed that palmitic acid (palm oil) and stearic acid (animal fat) showed a weak association with increases in risks for cardiovascular disease. A striking finding in these studies was that the presence of C-17 (heptadecanoic or margaric acid) was associated with a lower risk of heart disease (CHD). Thus, evidence has emerged that the beneficial effect of C-17) appears to present a favorable reduction of risks of CHD.

This situation links closely with the observations of the beneficial effects of C-17 in dolphins where the occurrence of Metabolic Syndrome is prevented by this saturated fat, (C-17, heptadecanoic acid). Of course, Metabolic Syndrome is a clear risk factor for CHD and the riddle of Metabolic Syndrome may be explained with C-17 (heptadecanoic acid) playing a pivotal role. These and other findings support, in part, the extrapolation of dolphin research to humans.

UNSATURATED FATS FAIL TO PROMOTE HEART HEALTH

An informative study concerning the inability of polyunsaturated omega 6 fatty acids to prevent CHD was published in the British Medical Journal on 4th February, 2013. (*www.bmj-press-releases/2013/02/04/study-raises-questions-about-dietary-fats-and-heart-disease-guidance*). In these studies, an in depth analysis of 458 men aged 30-59 years, who had recently had a heart attack or angina, showed that two groups of individuals (one with lower intake of saturated fats but increases of omega 6 fatty acid intake and one with no specific dietary advice) had major differences in death rates from cardiovascular disease and death from all causes.

The results of these latter studies showed that negative cardiovascular outcomes were more common in the omega 6 supplemented group compared with the control group (who had no specific dietary advice). Thus, omega 6 polyunsaturated fatty acids had negative health effects in the presence of a common belief that unsaturated fats may provide benefits in reductions of cardiovascular risks. While the lay reader may find some of this technical information hard to fathom, it is important for everyone to follow healthy heart guidelines regardless of fat intake. This can be achieved by engaging in regular exercise, avoidance of smoking, and watching dietary intakes of various foods, with reductions of salt and sugar intake, while selecting a dietary inclusion of healthy fruit and vegetables. These important lifestyle adjustments are important for heart health.

DAIRY FAT IMPROVES GLUCOSE TOLERANCE

Recent studies show that dairy fat (saturated) improves glucose tolerance. This circumstance is presumed to be due to improvements in insulin sensitivity and reductions in liver fat (*Kratz M et al Dairy fat intake is associated with glucose tolerance, hepatic and systemic insulin sensitivity, and liver fat but not beta-cell function Am.J.Clin Nutr. 2014, June; 99 (6) 1385-96).* The aim of these latter studies was to investigate whether or not dairy fat is associated with changes in glucose tolerance and factors that determine glucose tolerance. Lack of glucose tolerance is present in diabetes and may be abnormal in cases of insulin resistance (associated with the Metabolic Syndrome X).

In the quoted studies (*Kratz M. et al ibid, 2014*), changes in blood fats (lipids) were monitored. Among the findings was an inverse relationship between the saturated fatty acid C-17:0 (heptadecanoic acid) and glucose tolerance (and liver fat). This means that the presence of C-17 appeared to be associated with more beneficial effects on glucose tolerance (and liver fat). These findings support the belief that dairy fat, including C-17 may improve oral glucose tolerance (an anti-diabetic effect).

Furthermore, it has been found that dietary advice to change diary food intake does not appear to have a major effect on blood levels of fatty acids. However, studies have shown a significant beneficial effect of increased dairy intake on increasing C-17 (heptadecanoic acid) levels (*Benetar J A, Steward R A, The effects of changing dairy intake on trans and saturated fatty acid levels – results from a randomized controlled study, Nutr. J. 2014, Apr. 3; 13-32*). Among changes in other fats, this study (*Benetar et al ibid, 2014*) shows that extra consumption of dairy can raise heptadecanoic acid (C-17:0) levels by the consumption of about 3 daily servings of dairy food for one month.

MORE EVIDENCE THAT C-17 BENEFITS HUMAN METABOLIC SYNDROME

While heptadecanoic acid (C-17) deficiency seems to play a key role in the occurrence of Metabolic Syndrome X or a diabetes-like state in dolphins, it appears from some early studies that the same could be true in humans. Japanese researchers studied serum (blood) fatty acid and lipid concentrations in patients with and without Metabolic Syndrome X and found that C-15:0 and C-17:0 were lower in subjects with Metabolic Syndrome X, whereas specific C-20 fatty acids were higher (*Maruyama C et al Differences in serum phospholipid fatty acid compositions and estimated desaturase activities between Japanese men* with and without the metabolic syndrome *J.Atherosceler.Thromb.2008, Dec. 15 (6) 306-13*). These findings are consistent with the belief that C-17 plays a role in protection against Metabolic Syndrome X in humans.

DAIRY FAT AND HEART ATTACK

The evidence that milk fat intake does not increase the risk of a first myocardial infarction was demonstrated by Swedish researchers in 2004 (*Warensjo E et al Estimated intake of milk fat is negatively associated with cardiovascular risk factors and does not increase the risk of a first acute myocardial infarction. A prospective case-control study. Br. J. Nutr. 2004, Apr. 9, 1 (4): 635-42*). In this Swedish study, estimated milk fat intake was measured by serum testing of pentadecanoic acid (15:0) and heptadecanoic acid (C-17:0). These serum levels of fatty acids were negatively correlated with a number of cardiovascular and other risk factors, for example measures of insulin resistance. In other words, the higher the serum concentrations C-15 and C-17, the lower the presence of insulin resistance, but more important the lower the risk for a first ever heart attack (myocardial infarction). However, this apparent protection against the risk of coronary heart disease and the insulin resistance syndrome was removed when other clinical risk factors for heart attack were taken into consideration. These studies show that risks of heart disease or Metabolic Syndrome may have other causes in addition to just changes in serum fatty acids or blood fats. Disease causation in these circumstances appear to be multifactorial.

FATTY ACIDS, MORBIDITY AND MORTALITY

In elegant recent studies, the association between saturated fatty acid and trans-unsaturated fatty acid intake has been reviewed in relationship to all cause mortality, cardiovascular disease (CVD) and sequelae, coronary heart disease (CHD), ischemic stroke and type 11 diabetes mellitus (*de Souza R J et al, Intake of saturated and trans unsaturated fatty acids and risk of all cause mortality, cardiovascular disease, and type 11 diabetes: systemic review and meta-analysis of observational studies, BMJ, 2015; 351 doi: http://dx.doi.org/10.1136/bmj. h3978 Published 12 August 2015 cited as BMJ 2015; 351: h 3978*).

These latter studies showed that saturated fats are not associated with substantial changes in all cause mortality, CVD, CHD, ischemic stroke or type 11 diabetes. In contrast, transfats are associated with all cause mortality, total CHD, and CHD mortality.

Saturated fatty acids and trans-fats contribute to about 10 percent and 1-2 percent, respectively of energy in the U.S. diet. While some studies have shown modest improvements in the occurrence of CVD and CHD by reducing saturated fat intake, the benefits of the elimination of trans-fats are clear.

Dietary guidelines have recommended that saturated fats should be taken in limited amounts (less than 10 percent or 5-6 percent for individuals who need control of LDL (low density lipoprotein cholesterol levels) in the blood (*discussed in Souza R J et al (ibid, 2015)* Relevant to the present discussions in this booklet, Souza et al (*ibid, 2015*) uncovered studies that showed an inverse relationship between 16:1 n-7 trans-palmitoleic acid of dairy origin and type 11 diabetes (an antidiabetic effect).

It is notable that associations between red or processed meat (major sources of saturated fat) and the occurrence of type 11 diabetes exist (*Pan A et al Changes in red meat consumption and subsequent risk of Type 11 diabetes mellitus: three cohorts of U.S. men and women JAMA. Intern.Med 2013;173,1328-35*). In contrast, inverse associations have been reported for dairy products (an antidiabetic effect) (*Lee J E et al Meat intake and cause-specific mortality: a pooled analysis of Asian prospective cohort studies Am.J.Clin.Nutr.2013;98;1032-41*).

In a large case study of 12043 individuals, it was found that even chain fatty acids were associated with the incidence of type 11 diabetes, but odd chain fatty acids e.g. pentadecanoic and heptadecanoic acid were inversely associated with the presence of diabetes (a presumed anti-diabetic effect) (*Farouhi N G et al Differences in the prospective association between individual plasma phospholipid saturated fatty acids and incident Type 11 diabetes: the EPIC – Interact case cohort study Lancet Diabetes Endocrinol.2014;2:810-8*). In summary, odd chain saturated fatty acids are markers of dairy intake in the diet and even chain fatty acids are poor predictors of overall dietary intake.

The plot thickens as it becomes apparent that trans-palmitoleic acid could play a role in the prevention of type 11 diabetes mellitus. Dr. R J de Souza et al (*ibid 2015*) describes the association of trans-palmitoleic acid with diabetes prevention in a consistent manner in reviewed studies (*Souza R J, ibid, 2015*). Moreover, these researchers hypothesize that the protective effective of trans-palmitoleic acid may be a mimic of cis-palmitoleic acid which is known to protect against diabetes in animal models (*Cao H et al Identification of a lipokine, a lipid hormone linking adipose tissue to systemic metabolism.cell 2008; 134: 933-44*). Perhaps there is good reason to avoid blanket demonization of some saturated or trans-fats in the cause of diabetes.

PLANT PROTEIN DIETS CONFER HEALTH ADVANTAGES

There is a plethora of information in medical literature which reaches overall conclusions that switching from animal to plant protein-containing diets may improve health. A recent study has linked high levels of animal protein consumption in individuals under 65 years with risks of premature death (Levine, M.E., et al Low Protein Intake Is Associated with a Major Reduction in IGF, Cancer, and Overall Mortality in the 65 and Younger but Not Older Population, Cell Metabolism, 19, 407-417, 2014).

In these latter studies (*Levine et al ibid, 2014*) it is striking that the risks of premature death were considerably less when protein was of plant origin, notably beans and vegetables. The results of this study suggested that low animal protein intake during middle age, which is followed by moderate to high protein intake in the elderly, may improve longevity. The magnitude of the negative effects of preferential animal protein intake in these studies was highly significant. There was a four fold increase in the risk of death from cancer and diabetes and nearly two times the risk of dying from any cause over an eighteen year period of study. The risks of high animal protein intake were perceived as equivalent in harm to health problems caused by smoking, but arguments have prevailed because of the many difficulties in defining the health effects of individual nutrients by controlling for other factors that determine health and longevity.

In experimental animals, growth hormone receptor deficiency or growth hormone deficiency are known to prolong lifespan and reduce age-related degenerative diseases, including cancer and diabetes. In fact, humans with growth hormone receptor deficiency have decreased levels of IGF-1. These individuals have reduced cancer mortality and a lower prevalence of diabetes (*Levine M. E., et al, ibid, 2014*).

The dietary restriction of certain amino acids (methionine and tryptophan) may explain the effect, at least in part, on enhancing longevity and certain chronic disease risk. This dietary restriction of protein may result in lower IGF-1 levels and increase longevity with a reduction in the occurrence of cancer. These effects could be independent of calorie intake and they are further examples of the effects of protein selection (or dietary composition) on disease incidence and mortality.

The results of the epidemiological study of 6,381 men and women aged 50 years and above provide understanding of the links between dietary sources and amounts of protein intake, disease incidence, mortality and aging (*Levine, M.E., ibid, 2014*). It is apparent that the amount of protein of animal origin consumed accounted for a large proportion of the demonstrated association of total protein intake and all causes of mortality. It seems that high levels of protein intake that cause high levels of insulin and IGF-1 may be a key cause of mortality in individuals aged 50 to 65 years of age.

These recent studies (Levine, M.E., ibid, 2014) implied that low protein intake in elderly individuals (> 65 years of age) was detrimental. It has been reasoned that elevation of IGF-1 and insulin is beneficial in older subjects where weight tends to decline and sarcopenia occurs. Elderly subjects who have lost body weight as a consequence of aging are likely to be vulnerable to protein malnourishment. Genetic factors and co-existent diseases may amplify the negative effects of protein restriction in the elderly.

In summary, the studies of Levine, M.E. (ibid, 2014) imply that a reduced protein diet in middle age may be beneficial in cancer and diabetes prevention, with a decrease in overall mortality. This phenomenon may be related to a significant degree to the changes in circulating IGF-1 and insulin levels. These findings are supported by animal experiments in mice where high protein diets cause rises in IGF-1, which results in an increased risk of cancer. Several animal experiments and population studies indicate that diets rich in plant-based foods are likely to confer major health benefits in all adults. These conclusions are supported by several pivotal studies, listed below:

- Estruch, J. et al, N. Engl. J. Med., 2013, 368 1279-1290. These studies show the importance of a Mediterranean diet in the prevention of cardiovascular disease.
- Linos, E. and Willett, W.C., J. Natl. Compr. Cancer. Netw, 2007, 5, 711-718. This study shows the benefit of plant-based diets on breast cancer reduction.
- Michaud et al, Cancer Causes Control, 2001, 12, 557-567. This study links animal protein intake to prostate cancer occurrence.
- Willett, W.C., Public Health and Nutrition, 2006, 9, 1A, 105-110. This series of observations links the Mediterranean diet with health advantages.

AMPLIFYING THE EFFECTS OF C-17: ALPHA-LIPOID ACID

A number of dietary supplements have been proposed to be of particular value in the management of diabetes and Metabolic Syndrome X. Most notable among such supplements is alpha-lipoid acid. Alpha-lipoic acid is found in extracts of potatoes. In humans, this acid is synthesized in the liver and other tissues and engages as a natural co-factor in enzyme complexes, such as a key compound called pyruvate dehydrogenase. This enzyme is located in the cell in the mitochondria. In brief, alpha-lipoic acid plays a major role in the generation of energy from glucose metabolism in the powerhouses of the cell (the mitochondria). Moreover, alpha-lipoic acid functions as a powerful antioxidant that mops up damaging "free radicals". These free radicals are generated in large amounts in the mitochondria and they cause tissue damage by a mechanism of oxidative stress.

Many scientific studies show insulin resistance and diabetes are associated with the generation of damaging oxidative stress to tissues. This damage can result in diabetic complications. Moreover, oxidative stress can impact early stages of diabetes by promoting insulin resistance. In summary, alpha-lipoic acid can reduce oxidative stress and have positive effects on correcting insulin resistance and lowering blood glucose. The properties of alpha-lipoic acid make it an ideal candidate to act synergistically (in an additive manner) with heptadecanoic acid in the management of Metabolic Syndrome X (prediabetes) and diabetes mellitus.

SUPPLEMENTATION FOR DIABETES AND METABOLIC SYNDROME

In this monograph it has become apparent that the dietary supplementation of heptadecanoic acid may be valuable in both the management of Type 11 diabetes mellitus and Metabolic Syndrome X. This could be achieved by altered diet (selected addition of certain fish) or the use of a heptadecanoic acid-enriched dietary supplement. The evidence that mammalian (dolphin) cases of prediabetes or diabetes appears convincing where the switch of abnormal to normal glucose metabolism may be caused by the availability of heptadecanoic acid. Using sources of C-17 (heptadecanoic acid) as a supplement can be anticipated to be a safe process since this saturated fatty acid is established in the food chain.

Origins of heptadecanoic acid for supplement creation are found in high fat foods, especially butter with other dairy sources. In addition, C-17 is present in rye in relatively small amounts but it is conspicuous in shark liver oil, certain fish (e.g. mullet and mackerel) and beef fat (tallow). Of all other potential dietary supplements with benefits for diabetes and Metabolic Syndrome X, alpha lipoic acid has powerful beneficial effects on body metabolism. The addition of alpha-lipoic acid may be associated with clear benefits.

REFERENCES

Benetar, J A, Steward R A, The effects of changing dairy intake on trans and saturated fatty acid levels – results from a randomized controlled study, Nutr. J. 2014, Apr. 3; 13-32.

Cao H et al Identification of a lipokine, a lipid hormone linking adipose tissue to systemic metabolism.cell 2008; 134: 933-44.

Chowdhury, R. et al Association of Dietary, Circulating, and Supplement Fatty Acids with Coronary Risk: A systematic Review and Meta-analysis 18 March, 2014, Vol. 160. No.6: 398-406.doi:10.7326/M13-1788.

Chris.ramsden@nih.gov (research director) or Philip Calder at pcc@soton.ac.uk (editorial director), (accessed on the internet, July 29, 2015).

de Souza R J et al, Intake of saturated and trans unsaturated fatty acids and risk of all cause mortality, cardiovascular disease, and type 11 diabetes: systemic review and meta-analysis of observational studies, BMJ, 2015; 351 doi: http://dx.doi.org/10.1136/bmj. h3978 Published 12 August 2015 cited as BMJ 2015; 351: h 3978.

Farouhi N G et al Differences in the prospective association between individual plasma phospholipid saturated fatty acids and incident Type 11 diabetes: the EPIC – Interact case cohort study Lancet Diabetes Endocrinol.2014;2:810-8

Hal, Conick www.dairyreporter.com/Markets/Lack-ofdairy-based-fat-in-human-diet-mayleadto..., accessed 7/28/15.

Lee J E et al Meat intake and cause-specific mortality: a pooled analysis of Asian prospective cohort studies Am.J.Clin.Nutr.2013;98;1032-41.

Maruyama, C et al Differences in serum phospholipid fatty acid compositions and estimated desaturase activities between Japanese men with and without the metabolic syndrome J.Atherosceler.Thromb.2008, Dec. 15 (6) 306-13.

PLOS ONE, July 22, 2015. DOI 101371/journal pone 0132117 and
www.medicalexpress.com/news/2015-07-dolphins-diabetes-humans.html.

Venn-Watson S. K. et al Increased Dietary Intake of Saturated Fatty Acid
Heptadecanoic (C-17:0) Associated with Decreasing Ferritin and Alleviated
Metabolic Syndrome in Dolphins PLOS ONE, 2015; 10(7): e0132117 DOI; 10,
1371/journal pone 0132117.

www.bmj-press-releases/2013/02/04/study-raises-questions-about-dietary-fats-
and-heart-disease-guidance.

www.calacademy.org/explore-science/dolphins-Feb. 19, 2010, Science News
"Dolphins and Diabetes".

www.diabetes.co.uk/in-depth/every-last-shred-evidence-low-fat-dietary-
guidelines-..., accessed 7/28/2015).

www.nmmf.org/diabetes/metabolism/.

ABOUT THE AUTHOR

Dr. Stephen Holt is a best-selling author, medical practitioner in New York and Distinguished Professor of Medicine (Emeritus) at NYCPM. He has been described as a visionary, a pioneer of Integrative Medicine and is world-renowned for his work on therapeutics with nutrition and dietary supplements. He is a frequent guest lecturer at medical and scientific conferences.

Dr. Holt's principal training has been in allopathic medicine, but he has charted new treatment paradigms using natural medicines. He believes in the concept of "medical pluralism", where many different medical disciplines come together to provide holistic healthcare. Dr. Holt supports the practice of many forms of medicine including: chiropractic medicine, naturopathic medicine, podiatric medicine, homeopathic medicine, as well as traditional medical disciplines that offer many alternative strategies for health maintenance.

He is an author of more than 20 books in the popular healthcare field and he has also contributed chapters and many articles to peer-reviewed medical textbooks and journals. As well as publishing several hundred scientific articles in leading medical journals, Dr. Holt has been cited thousands of times in the medical and lay press.

An honors graduate in medicine from Liverpool University Medical School, in England, UK, Dr. Holt holds sub-specialty qualifications in gastroenterology and internal medicine in the USA, Canada and Europe. He has practiced clinical nutrition medicine for four decades. Dr. Holt has held the rank of full professor of medicine and bioengineering adjunct for many years and he has received awards for medical teaching and research, in the United States, China, Indonesia, Great Britain, Malaysia, Thailand, Taiwan, South Korea and other countries, where he has served as a Visiting Professor. He now holds the highest academic rank as a Distinguished Professor of Medicine (Emeritus).

OTHER BOOKS BY THE AUTHOR (Available for purchase at www.stephenholtmd.com)

Skinner HA, Holt S, The Alcohol Clinical Index, Addiction Research Foundation, Toronto, 1993

Holt S, Soya for Health, Mary Ann Liebert Publishers, Larchmont, NY 1996

Holt S, and Comac L, Miracle Herbs, Carol Publishing, Secaucus, NJ 1997

Holt S and Barilla J, The Power of Cartilage, Kensington Publishers, NY, NY 1998

Holt S, The Sexual Revolution, ProMotion Publishing, San Diego, California 1999

Holt S, The Natural Way to a Healthy Heart, M. Evans Inc., NY, NY 1999

(second printing 2002)

Holt S, The Soy Revolution, Dell Publishing, Random House, NY, NY, 1999 (third printing 2002)

Holt S, Natural Ways to Digestive Health, M. Evans Inc., NY, NY 2000 (second printing 2002)

Holt S and Bader D, Natures Benefit for Pets, Wellness Publishing, Newark, NJ 2001

Holt S, The Antiporosis Plan, Wellness Publishing, Newark, NJ 2002

Holt S, Combat Syndrome X, Y, and Z, Wellness Publishing, Newark, NJ 2002

Holt S, Wright J, Syndrome X Nutritional Factors, Wellness Publishing, Newark, NJ, 2003

Holt S, Enhancing Low Carb Diets, Wellness Publishing, Newark, NJ 2004

Holt S, Sleep Naturally, Wellness Publishing, Newark, NJ 2003

Holt S, Supreme Properties of Hoodia, Wellness Publishing, Newark, NJ 2005

Holt S, The HCG Diet Revolution, Authorhouse, Indiana, 2011 (www.authorhouse.com)

Holt S, The Antiaging Triad, Authorhouse, Indiana, 2011 (www.authorhouse.com)

Holt S, A Primer of Natural Therapeutics, Holt Institute of Medicine (2009) (www.stephenholtmd.com)

Holt S, Holt on: Sex The Natural Way, Authorhouse, Indiana, 2012 (www.authorhouse.com)

Holt S, A Definitive Guide to Colon Hydrotherapy", Creative Publishing Platform, 2014

Holt S, The Definitive Guide to Colon Hydrotherapy, Holt Institute of Medicine (2013). Creative Space Publishing Platform

Holt S, Nwosu U, Carroll C The Topical Pain Relief Revolution: Principles and Practice of Compounding Pharmacy, Holt Institute of Medicine, Creative Publishing Platform, 2014

Holt S, The Cannabis Revolution, Author House, 2015

www.ingramcontent.com/pod-product-compliance
Lightning Source LLC
Chambersburg PA
CBHW060708280326
41933CB00012B/2347